The Metabolism Connection:

Unlocking the Secrets of Boundless Energy.

By :

MAX HEWITT

Table of Contents.

Introduction

Metabolism is the intricate network of chemical processes that convert food into energy, playing a crucial role in our overall health. Understanding metabolism is vital, as it influences everything from weight management to energy levels and disease prevention. This book explores the profound connection between metabolism and energy, revealing how optimizing metabolic function can unlock boundless vitality.

Within these pages, you'll find actionable insights and practical strategies to enhance your metabolic health. Whether you're looking to improve your energy levels, manage your weight, or simply feel better, this guide will provide the tools you need for a healthier, more vibrant life. Let's embark on this journey to uncover the secrets of your metabolism and harness its power for lasting wellness.

Chapter 1: The Foundations of Metabolism

Defining Metabolism and Its Vital Role

Metabolism is a complex process that encompasses all the chemical reactions occurring within our bodies to maintain life. It's not just about how we burn calories; it's the foundation of our health, energy levels, and overall well-being. Metabolism can be divided into two main categories: catabolism and anabolism.

- **Catabolism** refers to the breakdown of molecules to obtain energy. For example, when we eat food, our body breaks down carbohydrates, proteins, and fats into simpler molecules that can be used for energy.

- **Anabolism**, on the other hand, is the process of building up larger molecules from smaller ones, such as the synthesis of proteins from amino acids.

These processes work together in a delicate balance, influencing how we grow, repair tissues, and respond to physical activity. Essentially, metabolism is the engine that drives our biological functions.

Understanding metabolism is crucial because it affects how efficiently our body utilizes energy. Factors such as age, gender, body composition, and genetics can influence metabolic rates, highlighting the unique aspects of each individual's metabolic health. Recognizing this can empower us to make informed decisions about our lifestyle and health.

How Metabolism Affects Energy and Health

The relationship between metabolism and energy is profound. Energy is derived from the food we consume, which is transformed through metabolic processes into a usable form primarily ATP (adenosine triphosphate). This energy fuels every action we take, from basic physiological functions like breathing and circulation to more complex activities like exercise and cognitive tasks.

When our metabolism functions optimally, we experience:

- **Sustained Energy Levels**: A well-functioning metabolism converts food into energy efficiently, preventing spikes and crashes in energy levels that can lead to fatigue.

- **Healthy Weight Management:** An effective metabolic rate helps maintain a healthy weight by balancing the energy we consume with the energy we expend.

- **Enhanced Physical Performance**: Metabolism supports muscle repair and growth, which is essential for anyone engaged in regular physical activity.

On the flip side, metabolic dysfunction can lead to a host of health issues. Conditions such as obesity, type 2 diabetes, and metabolic syndrome are directly linked to imbalances in metabolic processes. These conditions can arise from a sedentary lifestyle, poor diet, and hormonal changes, highlighting the need for awareness and proactive measures to promote metabolic health.

Essential Functions of Metabolic Processes

Metabolic processes play several vital roles in our bodies, beyond just energy production. Here are a few key functions:

1. **Nutrient Utilization:** Metabolism ensures that the nutrients from our food are effectively converted into energy and used for various bodily

functions. This process includes the breakdown of carbohydrates into glucose, fats into fatty acids, and proteins into amino acids.

2. **Hormonal Regulation:** Metabolism is closely linked to hormonal balance. Hormones like insulin, glucagon, and thyroid hormones regulate various metabolic pathways, influencing how our bodies process and store energy. For example, insulin facilitates the uptake of glucose into cells, helping to maintain stable blood sugar levels.

3. **Detoxification:** The liver, a key player in metabolism, helps detoxify harmful substances from our body. It converts toxins into harmless byproducts that can be excreted through urine or bile. A healthy metabolism supports the liver's ability to carry out these essential detoxification processes.

4. **Thermoregulation:** Metabolic processes also contribute to maintaining our body temperature. The energy produced through metabolism generates heat, which is crucial for keeping our internal environment stable, especially in varying external temperatures.

5. **Cellular Repair and Growth:** Metabolism provides the necessary energy and building blocks for cellular repair and growth. This is vital for recovery after injury, muscle building, and overall tissue maintenance.

Understanding these foundational aspects of metabolism empowers us to appreciate its role in our health. By fostering good metabolic practices such as a balanced diet, regular exercise, and adequate sleep we can unlock our body's potential for optimal energy and health. This book will delve deeper into these topics, providing insights and actionable strategies to enhance our metabolic function and, ultimately, our quality of life.

Chapter 2: Core Influences on Metabolic Health

Metabolic health is not determined by a single factor; rather, it is the result of a complex interplay among several core influences, with diet, sleep, and stress taking center stage. Each of these elements significantly impacts how our bodies metabolize food, regulate energy, and maintain overall health.

Diet: The Fuel for Metabolism

Diet is the cornerstone of metabolic health. What we eat directly affects how our bodies convert food into energy and how efficiently we use that energy. A balanced diet rich in whole foods, including fruits, vegetables, lean proteins, whole grains, and healthy fats, is essential for optimal metabolic function.

1.**Macronutrients and Their Roles:** Our diet consists of three main macronutrients: carbohydrates, proteins, and fats. Each plays a unique role in metabolism:

- **Carbohydrates** are the body's primary source of energy. They are broken down into glucose, which fuels our cells. However, excessive intake of refined carbs can lead to insulin resistance and metabolic dysfunction.

- **Proteins** are crucial for muscle repair and growth. They provide amino acids necessary for various metabolic processes, including the production of hormones and enzymes.

- **Fats**, particularly healthy fats from sources like avocados, nuts, and olive oil, support hormone production and cellular function. They also provide a dense source of energy.

2. **Quality Over Quantity**: It's not just about how much we eat, but what we eat. Diets high in processed foods, added sugars, and unhealthy fats can impair metabolic health. Conversely, nutrient-dense foods enhance our metabolic processes, support hormonal balance, and improve energy levels.

3. **Meal Timing and Frequency:** Research suggests that when we eat can be as important as what we eat. Intermittent fasting, for example, has gained popularity for its potential to improve insulin sensitivity and promote fat loss. However, individual preferences and lifestyles should guide meal timing strategies.

Sleep: The Unsung Hero of Metabolism

Sleep is often overlooked, yet it plays a critical role in metabolic health. Quality sleep is vital for recovery, hormonal regulation, and overall well-being. Lack of sleep can disrupt metabolic processes and lead to weight gain, increased cravings for unhealthy foods, and decreased energy levels.

1. **Hormonal Balance**: Sleep affects the balance of hormones that regulate appetite and metabolism. Ghrelin, known as the hunger hormone, increases with sleep deprivation, leading to increased appetite, while leptin, which signals satiety, decreases. This imbalance can contribute to overeating and weight gain.

2. **Impact on Insulin Sensitivity:** Chronic sleep deprivation can lead to insulin resistance, a precursor to type 2 diabetes. When we don't get enough sleep, our bodies become less effective at processing glucose, resulting in higher blood sugar levels and increased fat storage.

3. **Circadian Rhythms:** Our bodies operate on a circadian rhythm, a natural internal clock that regulates sleep-wake cycles and metabolic processes. Disrupting this rhythm through irregular sleep patterns, late-night eating, or

excessive screen time can negatively impact metabolism. Establishing a consistent sleep schedule and creating a sleep-friendly environment can enhance metabolic health.

Stress: The Metabolic Disruptor

Stress is another critical factor influencing metabolism. The body's response to stress involves the release of hormones like cortisol, which can have both short-term and long-term effects on metabolic health.

1. **Cortisol and Fat Storage:** Chronic stress leads to elevated cortisol levels, which can promote fat storage, particularly in the abdominal area. This "stress belly" is not only unsightly but also linked to a higher risk of metabolic diseases.

2. **Food Choices Under Stress**: When we're stressed, we often gravitate toward comfort foods that are high in sugar and fat. This emotional eating can create a vicious cycle, leading to weight gain and further stress about body image or health.

3. **Mind-Body Connection:** Managing stress through mindfulness practices, such as meditation, yoga, or deep-breathing exercises, can have positive effects on metabolic health.

These practices can help regulate cortisol levels, improve sleep quality, and promote healthier food choices.

Hormonal Health and Its Effect on Metabolism

Hormones are powerful chemical messengers that play a vital role in regulating metabolism. Understanding how hormones influence metabolic processes can empower individuals to make informed lifestyle choices that support their health.

Key Hormones Involved in Metabolism

1. **Insulin:** Produced by the pancreas, insulin is essential for regulating blood sugar levels. It facilitates the uptake of glucose into cells for energy and promotes the storage of excess glucose as fat. Insulin sensitivity is crucial for metabolic health; higher sensitivity means better glucose utilization and lower risk of type 2 diabetes.

2. **Thyroid Hormones:** The thyroid gland produces hormones that regulate the body's metabolic rate. An underactive thyroid (hypothyroidism) can lead to weight gain, fatigue, and sluggish metabolism, while an overactive thyroid

(hyperthyroidism) can cause weight loss and increased energy expenditure.

3. **Leptin and Ghrelin:** Leptin, produced by fat cells, signals fullness to the brain, while ghrelin, produced in the stomach, signals hunger. The balance of these hormones is critical for appetite regulation and energy balance. Disruptions in their signaling can lead to overeating and weight gain.

Factors Affecting Hormonal Balance

1. **Dietary Choices:** Certain foods can impact hormone production and sensitivity. For example, diets high in sugar can lead to insulin resistance, while diets rich in omega-3 fatty acids can improve leptin sensitivity.

2. **Physical Activity:** Regular exercise can help regulate hormonal balance. It increases insulin sensitivity, promotes the production of muscle-building hormones, and helps manage stress levels.

3. **Sleep Quality:** As discussed earlier, quality sleep is essential for maintaining hormonal balance. Sleep deprivation can disrupt the production of key hormones, leading to metabolic dysfunction.

Daily Habits That Shape Metabolic Efficiency

Metabolic efficiency is not solely determined by genetics; it can be influenced by daily habits and lifestyle choices. Small, consistent changes can lead to significant improvements in metabolic health.

1. Staying Active Throughout the Day

Incorporating physical activity into daily routines can boost metabolism. Simple habits like taking the stairs, walking during breaks, or engaging in household chores can increase overall energy expenditure. Aim for a mix of aerobic exercise, strength training, and flexibility workouts to support metabolic health.

2. Mindful Eating

Practicing mindful eating can improve awareness of hunger and fullness cues. This approach encourages individuals to savor their food, eat slowly, and pay attention to their body's signals. Mindful eating can help prevent overeating and promote healthier food choices.

3. Hydration

Staying hydrated is essential for optimal metabolic function. Water is involved in various metabolic processes, including digestion and nutrient absorption. Aim to drink enough water throughout the day to support metabolic health.

4. Limiting Processed Foods

Reducing the intake of processed foods, which are often high in added sugars, unhealthy fats, and artificial additives, can improve metabolic efficiency. Focus on whole, nutrient-dense foods that provide essential vitamins and minerals for optimal health.

5. Prioritizing Recovery

Rest and recovery are just as important as physical activity. Ensure you get enough quality sleep each night and allow your body to recover after intense workouts. Recovery practices like stretching, foam rolling, and yoga can enhance muscle recovery and support metabolic health.

6. Building a Support System

Having a support system can make a significant difference in maintaining healthy habits. Surround yourself with individuals who share similar health goals, whether through workout partners, online communities, or friends and family. Sharing your journey can provide motivation and accountability.

Conclusion

The interplay between diet, sleep, stress, hormonal health, and daily habits creates a complex web that influences metabolic health. By understanding these core influences, we can take proactive steps to improve our metabolic function, leading to increased energy levels, better weight management, and enhanced overall health. As we continue to explore the various facets of metabolism throughout this book, remember that small, consistent changes can have a profound impact on your health journey.

Chapter 3: Nutrition for a Robust Metabolism

Nutrition is a fundamental pillar of metabolic health. The food we consume not only provides the energy necessary for daily activities but also influences how effectively our bodies metabolize that energy. In this chapter, we will explore foods that fuel metabolic health, the importance of balanced macronutrients, and strategies for long-term metabolic support through diet.

Foods That Fuel Metabolic Health

Certain foods are particularly beneficial for metabolism, promoting energy production, supporting cellular functions, and enhancing overall health. Here are some key food groups and specific examples that can boost metabolic health:

1. Whole Grains

Whole grains are rich in fiber, vitamins, and minerals. They provide a slow and steady release of energy, which is essential for maintaining stable blood sugar levels. Examples of whole grains include:

- **Quinoa**: A complete protein that contains all nine essential amino acids, quinoa is also rich in fiber and various micronutrients, making it a perfect addition to any meal.

- **Brown Rice:** Unlike white rice, brown rice retains its bran and germ, providing more fiber and nutrients. It can help you feel full longer and is a great source of energy.

- **Oats:** Oats are high in soluble fiber, which can help lower cholesterol levels and stabilize blood sugar. Overnight oats or oatmeal can be a nutritious breakfast option.

2. Lean Proteins

Protein is crucial for metabolic health as it helps build and repair tissues, produces enzymes and hormones, and supports immune function. Good sources of lean protein include:

- **Chicken and Turkey**: These poultry options are low in fat and high in protein, making them ideal for muscle maintenance and growth.

- **Fish:** Fatty fish like salmon and mackerel are not only high in protein but also rich in omega-3 fatty acids, which have anti-inflammatory properties and support heart health.

- **Legumes:** Beans, lentils, and chickpeas are excellent plant-based protein sources that also provide fiber, helping to regulate blood sugar levels.

3. Healthy Fats

Contrary to popular belief, fats are essential for a healthy metabolism. They support hormone production and are a concentrated source of energy. Focus on incorporating healthy fats intakes such as:

- **Avocados**: Packed with monounsaturated fats, avocados are also rich in fiber and potassium. They can help reduce inflammation and improve heart health.

- **Nuts and Seeds:** Almonds, walnuts, flaxseeds, and chia seeds provide healthy fats, protein, and fiber, making them a great snack for sustained energy.

- **Olive Oil**: A staple of the Mediterranean diet, olive oil is rich in monounsaturated fats and antioxidants. It can enhance the flavor of dishes while supporting metabolic health.

4. Fruits and Vegetables

Fruits and vegetables are loaded with vitamins, minerals, and antioxidants that support overall health and metabolism. They are also high in water and fiber, which can aid in digestion and weight management. Key examples include:

- **Berries:** Blueberries, strawberries, and raspberries are rich in antioxidants and fiber. They can improve insulin sensitivity and support heart health.

- **Leafy Greens:** Spinach, kale, and Swiss chard are nutrient-dense foods that provide vitamins A, C, and K, along with iron and calcium. They can help reduce inflammation and promote metabolic function.

- **Cruciferous Vegetables:** Broccoli, cauliflower, and Brussels sprouts contain compounds that support liver function and detoxification, important for maintaining metabolic health.

5. Fermented Foods

Fermented foods promote gut health by introducing beneficial bacteria into the digestive system. A healthy gut microbiome is linked to better metabolism and weight management. Consider including:

- **Yogurt:** Rich in probiotics, yogurt can aid digestion and enhance nutrient absorption. Opt for plain, unsweetened varieties to avoid added sugars.

- **Sauerkraut and Kimchi:** These fermented vegetables are not only flavorful but also provide probiotics that support gut health and may improve metabolic processes.

- **Kefir:** This fermented dairy drink is packed with probiotics and can be a nutritious addition to smoothies or enjoyed on its own.

By incorporating fermented foods or any of the foods mentioned above into your diet, you may experience improved metabolic function, energy and overall well-being. However consult a health care professional before adding fermented foods or others as the case maybe, if you have digestive issues, allergies or medication interaction.

The Importance of Balanced Macronutrients

Achieving a balanced intake of macronutrient carbohydrates, proteins, and fats is vital for metabolic health. Each macronutrient plays a unique role in energy production, hormone regulation, and overall body function.

1. Carbohydrates: The Primary Energy Source

Carbohydrates are the body's main source of energy, particularly for high-intensity activities. However, the type and quality of carbohydrates consumed matter greatly:

- **Complex Carbohydrates:** Focus on whole, unprocessed carbohydrates like fruits, vegetables, legumes, and whole grains. These foods provide essential nutrients and fiber, which can help regulate blood sugar levels.

- **Limit Refined Carbohydrates:** Foods high in added sugars and refined grains can lead to spikes in blood sugar and insulin resistance. Reducing these foods can improve metabolic health.

2. Proteins: Building Blocks of Metabolism

Protein is essential for maintaining muscle mass, which plays a critical role in metabolism. More muscle means a higher resting metabolic rate, leading to more calories burned at rest.

- **Adequate Protein Intake**: Aim for a protein intake that aligns with your activity level and goals.

- **Protein Timing:** Distributing protein intake evenly across meals can enhance muscle protein synthesis. Consider incorporating a source of protein in each meal and snack

3. Fats: Essential for Hormonal Health

Healthy fats are crucial for hormone production and absorption of fat-soluble vitamins (A, D, E, and K). They also provide long-lasting energy, making them an essential component of a balanced diet.

- **Focus on Healthy Fats:** Prioritize sources of unsaturated fats, such as olive oil, avocados, and fatty fish, while limiting saturated and trans fats found in processed foods.

- **Mind Your Portions:** While fats are beneficial, they are calorie-dense. Be mindful of portion sizes to maintain a balanced caloric intake.

Strategies for Long-Term Metabolic Support through Diet

Building a diet that supports long-term metabolic health requires mindful planning and consistent habits. Here are some strategies to help you sustain a robust metabolism:

1. Plan Your Meals

Meal planning can help you stay on track with your nutritional goals. By preparing meals in advance, you can ensure a balanced intake of macronutrients and avoid the temptation of unhealthy convenience foods.

- **Batch Cooking:** Prepare large quantities of whole grains, proteins, and roasted vegetables that can be easily mixed and matched throughout the week.

- **Create Balanced Plates:** Aim for a balance of macronutrients in each meal. For example, a meal might include protein, carbohydrates, and vegetables.

2. Stay Hydrated

Hydration is often overlooked but plays a crucial role in metabolic health. Dehydration can impair energy levels and cognitive function, leading to decreased physical activity and poorer food choices.

- **Drink Water Throughout the Day:** Keep a water bottle handy and aim to drink water consistently.

- **Incorporate Hydrating Foods:** Many fruits and vegetables have high water content. Include items or fruits like high in water content to contribute to your hydration needs.

3. Monitor Portion Sizes

Being mindful of portion sizes can prevent overeating and support weight management. Using smaller plates, measuring portions, and being aware of hunger cues can help you eat more mindfully.

- **Listen to Your Body:** Pay attention to hunger and fullness signals. Eat slowly and savor each bite to better recognize when you're satisfied.

- **Avoid Distractions:** Eating while watching TV or working can lead to mindless eating. Aim to eat at the table and focus on your meal.

4. Practice Flexibility

While consistency is key, it's important to allow for flexibility in your diet. Strict dieting can lead to feelings of deprivation and may cause unhealthy relationships with food.

- **Enjoy Treats in Moderation:** Allow yourself occasional indulgences without guilt. A balanced approach to nutrition means enjoying a variety of foods.
- **Adapt to Your Body's Needs:** Be responsive to your body's changing needs, whether due to activity level, stress, or health changes. Adjust your diet accordingly.

5. Educate Yourself

Understanding the nutritional value of foods and how they affect your body can empower you to make informed choices.

- **Read Labels:** Familiarize yourself with food labels to understand the nutritional content and ingredients of the products you buy.
- **Seek Reliable Sources:** Stay informed about nutrition through reputable books, websites, and professionals. Knowledge is a powerful tool in achieving and maintaining metabolic health.

Conclusion

Nutrition is a vital component of metabolic health, influencing how our bodies process energy and maintain overall well-being. By focusing on nutrient-dense foods, balancing macronutrients, and adopting long-term dietary strategies, individuals can support robust metabolism and enhance their quality of life. In the following chapters, we will continue to explore practical steps and strategies for optimizing metabolic health, empowering you to take control of your well-being and vitality.

Chapter 4: Exercise and Its Metabolic Benefits

Exercise is a crucial component of maintaining a healthy metabolism. It influences how efficiently our bodies burn calories, utilize nutrients, and regulate hormones. In this chapter, we will delve into the different types of exercise that optimize metabolism, the mechanisms through which movement boosts energy at the cellular level, and how to create a sustainable fitness routine that fits seamlessly into your lifestyle.

Different Types of Exercise for Optimal Metabolism

Understanding the various types of exercise and their specific benefits is essential for developing an effective fitness regimen. Here, we will explore three primary categories of exercise: aerobic, anaerobic, and flexibility training.

1. Aerobic Exercise

Aerobic exercise, also known as cardiovascular exercise, involves continuous and rhythmic physical activity that increases heart rate and breathing. This type of exercise is vital for improving cardiovascular health and boosting metabolism.

Examples: Running, cycling, swimming, brisk walking, dancing, and group fitness classes.

Benefits:

- **Increases Caloric Burn:** Aerobic exercise enhances the body's ability to burn fat for fuel, helping with weight management and fat loss.

- **Improves Endurance:** Regular aerobic activity builds endurance, allowing you to perform daily tasks with greater ease and efficiency.

- **Enhances Heart Health:** This type of exercise strengthens the heart muscle, improving blood circulation and lowering the risk of cardiovascular diseases.

2. Anaerobic Exercise

Anaerobic exercise focuses on short bursts of intense activity that rely on energy sources stored in the muscles. This type of exercise is crucial for building strength, muscle mass, and metabolic rate.

Examples: Weight lifting, sprinting, high-intensity interval training (HIIT), and bodyweight exercises.

Benefits:

- **Increases Muscle Mass:** Building muscle through anaerobic exercise elevates resting metabolic rate (RMR), meaning your body burns more calories even at rest.

- **Boosts Strength and Power:** Strength training improves overall strength, enhances athletic performance, and helps prevent injuries.

- **Enhances Metabolic Flexibility:** Anaerobic exercise trains the body to switch between different energy sources efficiently, supporting metabolic health.

3. Flexibility and Balance Training

Flexibility and balance exercises are often overlooked but play a vital role in overall fitness. These activities help improve range of motion, reduce injury risk, and enhance coordination.

Examples: Yoga, Pilates, tai chi, and static stretching.

Benefits:

- **Improves Mobility:** Increased flexibility helps maintain proper movement patterns and joint health, reducing the risk of injury.

- **Supports Recovery:** Stretching and flexibility work can aid in recovery after intense workouts, promoting muscle relaxation and reducing soreness.

- **Enhances Mind-Body Connection:** Practices like yoga emphasize mindfulness and breathing, contributing to mental well-being and stress reduction, which indirectly supports metabolic health.

How Movement Boosts Energy at the Cellular Level

Physical activity impacts metabolism at a cellular level by promoting various physiological adaptations that enhance energy production and utilization.

1. Mitochondrial Function

Mitochondria are the powerhouse of cells, responsible for producing adenosine triphosphate (ATP), the primary energy currency of the body. Exercise stimulates mitochondrial biogenesis, leading to:

- **Increased ATP Production:** More mitochondria mean more energy production, allowing for greater endurance and performance during physical activities.

- **Improved Fat Oxidation:** Regular exercise enhances the ability of mitochondria to utilize fat as a fuel source, improving metabolic efficiency.

2. Insulin Sensitivity

Physical activity significantly affects insulin sensitivity, which is the body's ability to respond to insulin and effectively utilize glucose. Regular exercise leads to:

- **Enhanced Glucose Uptake:** Exercise increases the number of glucose transporters in muscle cells, allowing for more effective uptake of glucose from the bloodstream.

- **Reduced Risk of Insulin Resistance:** Improved insulin sensitivity helps lower the risk of developing type 2 diabetes and other metabolic disorders.

3. Hormonal Regulation

Exercise influences the release of various hormones that play crucial roles in metabolism, including:

- **Increased Growth Hormone Levels:** This hormone promotes muscle growth and fat loss, enhancing overall metabolic health.

- **Elevated Catecholamine Levels:** Hormones such as adrenaline and noradrenaline increase during exercise, stimulating fat breakdown and energy production.

4. Enhanced Blood Circulation

Movement promotes better blood flow throughout the body, delivering oxygen and nutrients to cells while aiding in the removal of metabolic waste. Benefits include:

- **Improved Nutrient Delivery:** Enhanced circulation supports muscle recovery and energy production by ensuring that cells receive the nutrients they need to function optimally.

- **Efficient Waste Removal:** Regular movement helps clear lactic acid and other byproducts of metabolism, reducing fatigue and improving recovery.

Creating a Sustainable Fitness Routine

Establishing a fitness routine that is sustainable and enjoyable is essential for long-term adherence and metabolic health. Here are some strategies to help you create a personalized fitness plan:

1. Set Clear and Achievable Goals

Begin by identifying your fitness goals. Whether it's losing weight, gaining muscle, increasing endurance, or improving flexibility, setting clear goals can provide direction and motivation.

- **SMART Goals:** Use the SMART criteria (Specific, Measurable, Achievable, Relevant, Time-bound) to create realistic and motivating fitness objectives. For example, instead of saying, "I want to exercise more," a SMART goal could be, "I will run for 30 minutes three times a week for the next month."

2. Choose Enjoyable Activities

Finding physical activities that you genuinely enjoy is crucial for maintaining consistency. Experiment with different forms of exercise to discover what you love, whether it's dancing, hiking, swimming, or group fitness classes.

- **Mix It Up:** Incorporate a variety of activities to keep things fresh and enjoyable. This not only prevents boredom but also challenges different muscle groups and improves overall fitness.

3. Incorporate Movement into Daily Life

In addition to structured workouts, find ways to integrate movement into your daily routine. Simple changes can have a significant impact on overall activity levels.

- **Take the Stairs:** Opt for stairs instead of elevators whenever possible.

- **Walk or Bike**: Use walking or biking for short trips instead of driving.

- **Active Breaks**: Take short breaks throughout the day to stretch or walk, especially if you have a sedentary job.

4. Establish a Routine

Consistency is key to reaping the metabolic benefits of exercise. Establish a regular workout schedule that fits your lifestyle and commitments.

- **Set a Regular Time:** Choose specific days and times for your workouts, treating them like important appointments.

- **Be Flexible:** While having a routine is essential, allow for flexibility when needed. Life can be unpredictable, and adapting your schedule can help maintain a positive relationship with exercise.

5. Listen to Your Body

Paying attention to your body's signals is crucial for avoiding injuries and ensuring long-term success. Recognize when to push yourself and when to rest.

- **Rest and Recovery**: Allow for adequate rest days and recovery time between intense workouts to prevent burnout and overtraining.

6. Seek Support and Accountability

Having a support system can make a significant difference in maintaining motivation and consistency. Consider involving friends, family, or fitness communities in your journey.

- **Workout Buddies:** Find a workout partner to share your fitness goals, encourage each other, and hold each other accountable.

- **Join Classes or Groups:** Participating in group fitness classes or community sports can foster a sense of belonging and motivation.

7. Track Your Progress

Monitoring your progress can help you stay motivated and make necessary adjustments to your routine. Keep track of your workouts, nutrition, and how you feel physically and mentally.

- **Use a Journal or App:** Documenting your workouts and nutrition can help you identify patterns, celebrate achievements, and set new goals.
- **Regular Assessments:** Periodically assess your progress toward your goals, adjusting your routine as needed to continue challenging yourself.

Conclusion

Exercise is a powerful tool for enhancing metabolic health. By incorporating various types of exercise into your routine, understanding how movement boosts energy at the cellular level, and creating a sustainable fitness plan, you can significantly improve your overall health and well-being. In the following chapters, we will continue to explore additional aspects of metabolic health and how to support your body in achieving optimal performance and vitality.

Chapter 5: The Mind-Body Connection

The relationship between the mind and body is intricate and profound, influencing our overall health and well-being. One of the most significant areas where this connection manifests is in metabolism. In this chapter, we will explore how mental health affects metabolic processes, the interplay between stress and hormones in metabolic balance, and the importance of building resilience for maintaining both mental and physical vitality.

The Impact of Mental Health on Metabolism

Mental health significantly influences various physiological processes, including metabolism. A balanced mental state is essential for optimal metabolic function, while mental health issues can disrupt these processes and lead to negative health outcomes.

1. The Role of Emotions in Metabolism

Our emotions play a critical role in how our bodies metabolize food and energy. For instance:

- **Negative Emotions and Cravings:** Stress, anxiety, and depression can lead to emotional eating, resulting in cravings for high-calorie, low-nutrient foods. This can contribute to weight gain and metabolic syndrome.

- **Positive Emotions and Healthy Choices:** Conversely, positive emotions can encourage healthier food choices and motivate physical activity, supporting better metabolic health.

2. Mental Health Disorders and Metabolic Disturbances

Various mental health disorders can have profound effects on metabolism:

- **Depression:** This condition is often associated with changes in appetite and energy levels. Some individuals may experience weight gain due to overeating, while others may lose weight due to reduced appetite. Both scenarios can negatively impact metabolic health.

- **Anxiety:** Chronic anxiety can lead to increased cortisol levels, which may promote fat storage, particularly in the abdominal area, leading to obesity and related metabolic issues.

- **Bipolar Disorder:** Individuals with bipolar disorder may experience significant fluctuations in weight during manic and depressive episodes, affecting overall metabolic balance.

3. Neurotransmitters and Metabolism

The brain's chemistry plays a vital role in regulating appetite and energy expenditure. Key neurotransmitters involved in these processes include:

- **Serotonin**: Often referred to as the "feel-good" hormone, serotonin helps regulate mood and appetite. Low levels of serotonin can lead to increased cravings for carbohydrates and unhealthy foods.

- **Dopamine:** This neurotransmitter is associated with reward and pleasure. Dysregulation of dopamine can lead to changes in eating behavior and energy expenditure, affecting metabolism.

4. The Gut-Brain Connection

Emerging research has highlighted the connection between gut health and mental well-being, known as the gut-brain axis. The state of the gut microbiome can influence mental health, and vice versa:

- **Gut Microbiota and Mood:** A healthy gut microbiome produces neurotransmitters that can positively impact mood and mental health, promoting better metabolic function.

- **Inflammation:** An imbalance in gut bacteria can lead to inflammation, which is associated with various metabolic disorders, including obesity and insulin resistance.

Stress and Hormones in Metabolic Balance

Stress is a natural response to challenges and threats, but chronic stress can have detrimental effects on metabolism. Understanding the relationship between stress and hormones is crucial for maintaining metabolic balance.

1. The Stress Response

When faced with stress, the body activates the "fight or flight" response, releasing hormones such as adrenaline and cortisol. These hormones prepare the body to respond to immediate threats by increasing heart rate and energy availability.

- **Short-Term vs. Long-Term Stress:** Acute stress can enhance metabolic function by increasing energy availability; however, chronic stress leads to sustained high levels of cortisol, which can disrupt metabolic processes.

2. Cortisol and Its Effects on Metabolism

Cortisol, often called the "stress hormone," plays a crucial role in various metabolic processes:

- **Glucose Metabolism:** Cortisol increases blood sugar levels by stimulating gluconeogenesis (the production of glucose from non-carbohydrate sources). While this is beneficial in the short term, chronic elevation can lead to insulin resistance and diabetes

- **Fat Storage:** Prolonged cortisol exposure is associated with increased fat accumulation, particularly in the abdominal area. This type of fat is metabolically active and linked to a higher risk of metabolic diseases.

3. Hormonal Imbalances and Metabolic Health

Stress can disrupt the balance of other hormones that regulate metabolism:

- **Insulin:** Chronic stress can lead to insulin resistance, making it more difficult for the body to regulate blood sugar levels effectively.

- **Thyroid Hormones:** Stress can impair thyroid function, leading to decreased metabolism and weight gain. The thyroid gland regulates energy production, and any imbalance can affect overall metabolic health.

4. Strategies for Managing Stress

Managing stress effectively is crucial for maintaining metabolic balance. Here are some strategies to consider:

- **Mindfulness and Meditation:** Practicing mindfulness and meditation can reduce stress levels, improve emotional well-being, and support metabolic health.

- **Physical Activity**: Regular exercise is an effective way to manage stress and improve mood, which can positively impact metabolism.

- Social Support: Building strong social connections and seeking support from friends and family can help reduce stress and improve mental health.

Building Resilience for Mental and Physical Vitality

Resilience is the ability to adapt and bounce back from challenges. Building resilience is essential for maintaining both mental and physical vitality, supporting optimal metabolic health.

1. Understanding Resilience

Resilience involves a combination of mental, emotional, and physical strengths that allow individuals to cope with adversity effectively. Key components of resilience include:

- **Optimism:** Maintaining a positive outlook can enhance resilience and improve overall well-being.

- **Emotional Regulation:** The ability to manage and respond to emotions in a healthy way contributes to resilience.

- **Problem-Solving-Skills:** Developing effective problem-solving skills can help individuals navigate challenges more effectively.

2. Strategies for Building Resilience

Several strategies can help individuals build resilience and improve mental and physical vitality:

- **Self-Care Practices:** Prioritizing self-care activities such as exercise, proper nutrition, and adequate sleep is essential for maintaining resilience and overall health.

- **Goal Setting:** Setting realistic and achievable goals can provide a sense of purpose and motivation, fostering resilience.

- **Mindfulness Practices:** Engaging in mindfulness practices can enhance self-awareness and emotional regulation, contributing to greater resilience.

3. The Role of Community and Support Systems

Social connections and support systems play a vital role in building resilience:

- **Community Engagement:** Being part of a community can provide a sense of belonging and support, helping individuals navigate challenges more effectively.

- **Seeking Help:** Recognizing when to seek professional help for mental health issues is crucial. Therapists and counselors can provide valuable tools and strategies for building resilience.

4. The Synergy of Mind and Body

Ultimately, the mind-body connection is about recognizing that mental and physical health are intertwined. By nurturing both aspects, individuals can achieve greater resilience and improved metabolic health.

- **Holistic Approach:** Embracing a holistic approach to health that considers both mental and physical well-being can lead to better overall outcomes.

- **Positive Lifestyle Choices:** Making positive lifestyle choices, such as engaging in regular physical activity, eating a balanced diet, and prioritizing mental health, can significantly enhance both resilience and metabolism.

Conclusion

The mind-body connection is a powerful determinant of metabolic health. Understanding how mental health, stress, and resilience influence metabolism is essential for achieving optimal health. By fostering positive mental health, managing stress effectively, and building resilience, individuals can enhance their overall well-being and support a robust metabolism. In the following chapters, we will continue to explore additional aspects of metabolic health, providing practical strategies for maintaining vitality and energy throughout life.

Chapter 6: Aging and Metabolism

Aging is an inevitable part of life that profoundly affects every aspect of our being, including our metabolic processes. As we age, our bodies undergo significant changes that can impact our energy levels, overall health, and nutritional needs. This chapter will explore the complex relationship between aging and metabolism, focusing on how metabolic shifts occur with age, strategies to maintain energy and health over time, and the nutritional needs that arise from an aging metabolism.

Understanding Metabolic Shifts with Age

As we age, our metabolism undergoes a series of changes that can affect how our bodies utilize energy. Metabolism refers to all the biochemical processes that occur within our bodies to maintain life, including the conversion of food into energy. This process can slow down due to various factors:

1. **Declining Muscle Mass:** One of the most significant shifts in metabolism as we age is the

loss of lean muscle mass, a condition known as sarcopenia. Muscle tissue is metabolically active and plays a crucial role in burning calories. With less muscle, the resting metabolic rate (RMR) decreases, leading to fewer calories burned throughout the day.

2. **Hormonal Changes:** Aging is often accompanied by changes in hormone levels, including declines in testosterone, estrogen, and growth hormone. These hormonal shifts can lead to increased fat accumulation, particularly visceral fat, which is associated with various health risks, including cardiovascular disease and type 2 diabetes.

3. **Decreased Insulin Sensitivity:** As we age, our bodies may become less sensitive to insulin, a hormone critical for regulating blood sugar levels. This reduced sensitivity can result in higher blood sugar levels and an increased risk of metabolic disorders.

4. **Changes in Energy Expenditure:** The amount of energy expended during physical activity and at rest can also decline with age. Older adults tend to be less physically active, which contributes to a lower overall energy expenditure.

5. **Altered Nutrient Absorption:** Aging can impact the gastrointestinal system, leading to changes in nutrient absorption. The efficiency with which our bodies absorb nutrients from food can diminish, affecting overall health and energy levels.

Understanding these metabolic shifts is crucial for developing strategies to combat age-related metabolic decline. Recognizing that metabolism is not a static process empowers individuals to make informed choices that can enhance their health as they age.

Strategies to Maintain Energy and Health Over Time

Maintaining energy and health as we age requires a multifaceted approach that includes lifestyle modifications, physical activity, and dietary changes. Here are several strategies to consider:

1. **Incorporate Strength Training:** Engaging in regular strength training exercises is one of the most effective ways to combat muscle loss and boost metabolism. Resistance training helps to build and maintain muscle mass, thereby increasing RMR and enhancing overall metabolic function. Aim for at least two sessions of strength

training per week, focusing on all major muscle groups.

2. **Stay Active:** In addition to strength training, maintaining an active lifestyle is vital for metabolic health. Incorporate aerobic exercises such as walking, swimming, or cycling into your routine. Aim for moderate-intensity aerobic activity each week to support cardiovascular health and improve metabolic function.

3. **Prioritize Sleep:** Quality sleep is essential for metabolic health. Sleep deprivation can lead to hormonal imbalances that negatively affect metabolism, appetite regulation, and energy levels. Aim for quality sleep each night and establish a consistent sleep routine to support optimal metabolic health.

4. **Manage Stress:** Chronic stress can disrupt hormonal balance, particularly cortisol levels, which can negatively impact metabolism. Incorporate stress-reducing practices into your daily routine, such as mindfulness meditation, yoga, or deep-breathing exercises. These practices can help regulate stress hormones and promote overall well-being.

5. **Eat a Balanced Diet:** A nutrient-dense diet rich in whole foods is crucial for supporting

metabolism and overall health. Focus on consuming a variety of fruits, vegetables, whole grains, lean proteins, and healthy fats. Pay attention to portion sizes and avoid excessive intake of processed foods, sugars, and unhealthy fats.

6. **Stay Hydrated:** Proper hydration is often overlooked but is essential for optimal metabolic function. Water plays a critical role in digestion, nutrient absorption, and the elimination of waste products. Aim to drink enough water throughout the day, adjusting your intake based on activity level and environmental conditions.

7. **Regular Health Screenings:** As you age, regular health screenings become increasingly important. Monitoring blood pressure, cholesterol levels, blood sugar, and hormonal levels can help detect potential health issues early and guide necessary lifestyle changes.

8. **Consider Nutritional Supplements:** While a balanced diet should provide most of your nutritional needs, certain supplements may be beneficial as you age. Consult with a healthcare professional to determine if specific supplements, such as vitamin D, omega-3 fatty acids, or probiotics, could support your metabolic health.

By adopting these strategies, individuals can significantly improve their energy levels, health, and overall quality of life as they age. Taking proactive steps to maintain metabolic health is crucial for longevity and well-being.

Nutritional Needs for an Aging Metabolism

As metabolism shifts with age, so too do our nutritional needs. Understanding these changes can help individuals make informed dietary choices that support metabolic health:

1. **Increased Protein Intake:** With the decline in muscle mass, it is essential to consume adequate protein to support muscle maintenance and repair. Aim for high-quality protein sources such as lean meats, fish, eggs, dairy, legumes, and nuts. Incorporating protein in every meal can help preserve muscle mass and support metabolic function.

2. **Focus on Healthy Fats:** Healthy fats, such as those found in avocados, nuts, seeds, and olive oil, are crucial for brain health and hormone production. Incorporating these fats into your diet

can support overall health and provide sustained energy.

3. **Fiber-Rich Foods:** As metabolism slows, fiber becomes increasingly important for digestive health. Consuming a diet rich in fiber can help regulate blood sugar levels, improve satiety, and promote healthy bowel function. Aim to include plenty of fruits, vegetables, whole grains, and legumes in your meals.

4. **Antioxidant-Rich Foods:** Aging is associated with increased oxidative stress, which can contribute to various health issues. Foods rich in antioxidants, such as berries, leafy greens, and dark chocolate, can help combat oxidative damage and support overall health.

5. **Limit Processed Foods and Added Sugars:** Processed foods and added sugars can lead to weight gain and metabolic dysfunction. Focus on whole, minimally processed foods to support a healthy metabolism and overall well-being.

6. **Stay Mindful of Caloric Intake:** As metabolism slows, it becomes important to be mindful of caloric intake. While maintaining a balanced diet, ensure that portion sizes are appropriate for your energy needs. This can help prevent unwanted weight gain associated with aging.

7. **Hydration Considerations:** Older adults may have a diminished sense of thirst, making hydration more critical. Ensure adequate water intake throughout the day, especially when consuming higher levels of protein or engaging in physical activity.

8. **Individualized Nutrition Plans:** Since everyone's metabolic needs are different, it is essential to consider personalized nutrition plans that cater to individual health goals, preferences, and conditions. Consulting with a registered dietitian can help tailor a dietary approach that best supports metabolic health.

Conclusion

Understanding the intricate relationship between aging and metabolism is vital for promoting long-term health and vitality. By recognizing the metabolic shifts that occur with age and implementing strategies to maintain energy and health, individuals can take proactive steps toward supporting their well-being. Additionally, addressing the unique nutritional needs that arise from an aging metabolism can empower individuals to make informed dietary choices that enhance their quality of life. By focusing on these key aspects, individuals can unlock the potential for a healthier, more vibrant life as they age.

Chapter 7: The Role of Circadian Rhythms in Metabolic Health

Our bodies operate on an intricate clock known as the circadian rhythm, a natural, internal process that regulates the sleep-wake cycle and various physiological functions over a 24-hour period. Understanding how these rhythms influence our metabolism is crucial for optimizing health and well-being. This chapter will delve into the science behind circadian rhythms and energy, the relationship between sleep quality and metabolic function, and strategies for aligning lifestyle with these natural rhythms.

The Science of Circadian Rhythm and Energy

Circadian rhythms are driven by an internal clock located in the suprachiasmatic nucleus (SCN) of the brain. This clock synchronizes with environmental cues, primarily light, and darkness, allowing our bodies to anticipate changes in day and night. These rhythms influence various biological processes, including hormone release, sleep patterns, body temperature, and metabolism.

Hormonal Regulation: Circadian rhythms play a critical role in the regulation of hormones that directly affect metabolism. For instance, insulin, the hormone responsible for regulating blood sugar levels, exhibits a circadian pattern, with sensitivity fluctuating throughout the day. This means that our bodies process carbohydrates and sugars more efficiently at certain times than others. Disruption to these rhythms can impair insulin sensitivity and increase the risk of metabolic disorders like obesity and type 2 diabetes.

Metabolic Rate: Research shows that our resting metabolic rate (RMR) also varies throughout the day. Typically, metabolic rate is highest during the daytime, aligning with periods of activity and food intake, and declines in the evening as the body prepares for rest. This rhythm ensures that energy is utilized efficiently according to our daily activities and needs.

Energy Balance: The interaction between circadian rhythms and energy balance is complex. When circadian rhythms are aligned with our daily routines such as eating during daylight hours and sleeping at night our bodies function optimally. Conversely, misalignment, often seen in shift workers or those with irregular sleep schedules, can lead to dysregulation of hunger hormones (like ghrelin and leptin), increased appetite, and ultimately weight gain.

The Impact of Light Exposure: Light is a primary cue for regulating circadian rhythms. Exposure to natural light during the day helps maintain a healthy rhythm, while excessive artificial light exposure at night, particularly blue light from screens, can disrupt these patterns. This disruption can hinder melatonin production, a hormone that promotes sleep, leading to poor sleep quality and metabolic disturbances.

The Gut Microbiome: Emerging research suggests that circadian rhythms also influence the composition and function of the gut microbiome, the community of bacteria living in our digestive tract. These microorganisms play a vital role in metabolism, and their activity varies according to the time of day. Disruptions in circadian rhythms can alter microbiome diversity and function, potentially leading to metabolic issues such as obesity and metabolic syndrome.

By understanding the science behind circadian rhythms, individuals can make informed decisions to align their lifestyles with these natural cycles, optimizing energy use and supporting metabolic health.

Sleep Quality and Metabolic Function

Sleep is a cornerstone of metabolic health, and its quality and quantity can significantly impact our metabolic processes. The relationship between sleep and metabolism is bidirectional, where poor sleep can disrupt metabolic function and metabolic dysfunction can impair sleep quality.

The Role of Sleep in Metabolism: Sleep is essential for various metabolic processes, including glucose metabolism, fat storage, and appetite regulation. During sleep, the body undergoes repair and recovery, releasing growth hormones and regulating other hormones involved in metabolism. Lack of adequate sleep can lead to increased insulin resistance, making it more challenging for the body to utilize glucose effectively.

Hormonal Imbalances: Sleep deprivation affects the balance of hunger-related hormones. Ghrelin, the hormone that stimulates appetite, tends to increase when sleep is inadequate, while leptin, which signals satiety, decreases. This imbalance can lead to increased hunger, cravings for unhealthy foods, and weight gain over time.

Inflammation and Stress: Poor sleep quality is associated with elevated levels of inflammatory markers in the body. Chronic inflammation can contribute to insulin resistance and other metabolic disorders.

Additionally, inadequate sleep can elevate cortisol levels, the body's stress hormone, which further exacerbates metabolic dysregulation.

Cognitive Function and Decision Making: Sleep deprivation can impair cognitive function, making it more challenging to make healthy food choices and maintain a balanced diet. Individuals who are sleep-deprived may be more prone to cravings for high-calorie, processed foods, leading to poor dietary choices that can affect metabolism.

Sleep Disorders and Metabolic Health: Conditions such as sleep apnea, which disrupt sleep quality, are linked to metabolic syndrome and obesity. Addressing these sleep disorders is crucial for improving metabolic health and reducing the risk of associated conditions.

To promote metabolic health, it is essential to prioritize sleep hygiene. This includes creating a consistent sleep schedule, ensuring a dark and quiet sleep environment, and limiting exposure to screens before bedtime. By improving sleep quality, individuals can support their metabolic processes and enhance overall health.

Aligning Lifestyle with Natural Rhythms

To optimize metabolic health, it is vital to align lifestyle choices with circadian rhythms. Here are several strategies for harmonizing daily activities with these natural rhythms:

Establish a Consistent Sleep Schedule: Aim to go to bed and wake up at the same time every day, even on weekends. This consistency helps regulate the body's internal clock and can improve sleep quality and metabolic function.

Optimize Light Exposure: Maximize exposure to natural light during the day, particularly in the morning. This helps reinforce the circadian rhythm and boosts mood and energy levels. Conversely, minimize exposure to bright screens and artificial light in the evening to promote melatonin production and improve sleep quality.

Eat According to Your Body Clock: Timing of meals can significantly impact metabolism. Aim to consume most of your calories during daylight hours, aligning with the body's natural digestive rhythms. Avoid late-night eating, as this can disrupt metabolic processes and lead to weight gain.

Incorporate Physical Activity: Exercise can enhance circadian rhythms and improve sleep quality. Aim to engage in physical activity during the day, ideally in the morning or early afternoon, to support energy levels and promote a better night's sleep.

Practice Relaxation Techniques: Incorporating relaxation techniques into your evening routine, such as mindfulness, meditation, or gentle yoga, can help signal to the body that it is time to wind down. This can promote better sleep quality and improve metabolic health.

Monitor Caffeine and Alcohol Intake: Caffeine and alcohol can disrupt sleep patterns and circadian rhythms. Limit caffeine consumption in the afternoon and evening, and be mindful of alcohol intake, particularly close to bedtime.

Listen to Your Body: Pay attention to your body's natural cues for hunger, fatigue, and energy levels. Learning to recognize and respond to these signals can help you make choices that align with your circadian rhythms.

Prioritize Mental Health: Chronic stress can disrupt circadian rhythms and negatively impact metabolic health. Incorporating stress management techniques, such as journaling, spending time in nature, or engaging in hobbies, can help support mental well-being and promote healthier metabolic function.

Conclusion

Understanding the role of circadian rhythms in metabolic health is crucial for optimizing overall well-being. By recognizing the scientific principles behind these rhythms and their impact on energy, sleep quality, and lifestyle choices, individuals can make informed decisions that enhance their metabolic health. Prioritizing sleep, aligning daily routines with natural rhythms, and adopting healthy lifestyle practices can promote better metabolic function, energy levels, and long-term health. By embracing the power of circadian rhythms, individuals can unlock their potential for a healthier, more vibrant life.

Chapter 8: Metabolic Myths and Misconceptions

In the pursuit of better metabolic health, misconceptions can cloud effective strategies, leading to confusion and unrealistic expectations. This chapter aims to debunk prevalent myths, offer clarity on popular diet trends, and highlight ways to avoid common pitfalls in the quest for a healthy metabolism.

Separating Fact from Fiction: Common Myths

Metabolism is frequently misunderstood, leading to practices that may be ineffective or counterproductive. One of the most common myths is that a faster metabolism automatically equates to easier weight management. While metabolic rate does play a role in energy expenditure, it's just one aspect of a complex system influenced by genetics, lifestyle, and overall physical activity. Relying on extreme diets or supplements to boost metabolism often overlooks this multifaceted reality.

Another misconception is that skipping meals can jumpstart metabolism. In fact, this can slow down metabolic rate over time as the body adjusts to perceived scarcity by conserving energy. Consuming balanced, consistent meals better supports metabolic function and energy levels.

Exercise is another area surrounded by myths, with many assuming it alone can dramatically alter metabolic rate. While physical activity, particularly strength training, does increase resting metabolic rate through muscle gain, a well-rounded approach including balanced nutrition and lifestyle adjustments is key for meaningful metabolic improvement. Additionally, although aging influences metabolism, lifestyle choices play a powerful role in shaping metabolic health, often more so than age alone.

Finally, many believe that metabolism solely pertains to calorie burning. While it's true that metabolism involves energy expenditure, it's also central to other functions such as growth, repair, and hormone regulation. Understanding metabolism in this comprehensive way promotes a healthier, more sustainable approach to wellness.

The Truth Behind Some Diet Practice.

Popular diets frequently claim to optimize metabolism, yet their promises can be misleading or unsustainable. Rather than focusing on restrictive or one-size-fits-all plans, a balanced approach tailored to individual needs is typically more effective.

High-fat, low-carbohydrate diets, for example, are widely known and can result in temporary weight loss. However, their long-term effects on metabolic and overall health remain uncertain, and these diets may encourage unhealthy eating habits. Intermittent eating patterns, too, can offer benefits for some but may not be suitable for everyone, as they can lead to erratic eating habits.

Low-calorie diets also promise rapid results but may reduce metabolic rate over time, making it harder to maintain weight loss. Adopting a gradual, balanced approach is more beneficial for sustainable results. Likewise, plant-based diets can support metabolic health but need careful planning to avoid nutrient deficiencies, which could otherwise impact metabolism.

Lastly, detox diets, which claim to clear toxins and reset metabolism, overlook the body's natural detox systems like the liver and kidneys. Supporting these systems with a balanced, whole-food diet and adequate hydration is generally more effective than restrictive cleanses.

Avoiding Pitfalls in Pursuit of Metabolic Health

To navigate the abundance of metabolic health information, a holistic, evidence-based approach is essential. Fad diets or extreme methods can often cause more harm than good, so aiming for a well-rounded, balanced plan is key.

Prioritizing a diet rich in whole foods fruits, vegetables, whole grains, lean proteins, and healthy fats supports metabolic health with essential nutrients. Setting realistic, incremental goals rather than aiming for rapid changes helps ensure consistency and long-term benefits. Emphasizing total wellness over weight loss can bring additional benefits like improved mood, physical performance, and energy levels.

Exercise should be regular yet sustainable, focusing on enjoyable activities to encourage adherence. Combining strength training, cardiovascular workouts, and flexibility exercises promotes metabolic health. Additionally, prioritizing sleep and stress management is vital, as sleep influences hormonal regulation, and chronic stress can disrupt metabolic processes.

Developing relaxation and mindfulness practices can help regulate stress and improve sleep quality.

Finally, adopting a holistic perspective that incorporates mental and emotional well-being into health routines is essential. Building a supportive environment that promotes positive habits and addresses issues like emotional eating or body image can enhance metabolic health in sustainable ways.

In summary, separating fact from fiction, understanding popular diet trends, and adopting a balanced, comprehensive approach to health can empower individuals to make choices that truly support metabolic well-being. By embracing these strategies, readers can work toward improved overall health that's achievable and enduring.

Chapter 9: Environmental and Lifestyle Resilience

Environmental and lifestyle factors significantly impact metabolic health. Modern life presents unique challenges to maintaining a healthy metabolism due to environmental toxins, pollutants, stress, and lifestyle pressures that can disrupt our metabolic functions. This chapter explores how the environment affects metabolic health, offers ways to build resilience to external stressors, and provides practical lifestyle tips for fostering a healthier, more resilient metabolic state.

How Environment Affects Metabolic Health

Our environment, the air we breathe, the water we drink, the places we live and work plays a fundamental role in our overall health, particularly our metabolic processes. Numerous environmental factors influence metabolic health, some of which we might not initially associate with metabolism, but which significantly affect how our bodies function and respond.

Exposure to Toxins and Pollutants

Toxins and pollutants are a growing concern for metabolic health. Air pollution, for instance, is filled with particulate matter, heavy metals, and chemicals that, when inhaled, enter the bloodstream and can cause systemic inflammation. This inflammation triggers metabolic stress, leading to conditions such as insulin resistance, impaired fat metabolism, and other issues related to energy processing and utilization. Additionally, pollutants found in household products, plastics, and pesticides can act as endocrine disruptors, interfering with hormone function, including those related to metabolic regulation like insulin and cortisol.

Food Quality and Chemical Exposure

The quality of food and the presence of chemicals in our diet directly impact metabolic health. Processed foods often contain preservatives, artificial colors, and additives, which, over time, may disrupt the gut microbiome and, in turn, influence metabolism. Similarly, exposure to chemicals like pesticides and herbicides in non-organic produce can affect metabolic health, as some of these chemicals are associated with obesity, insulin resistance, and metabolic disorders.

Lack of Sunlight and Vitamin D Deficiency

Exposure to natural sunlight is crucial for the body to produce vitamin D, a hormone essential for metabolic health. Vitamin D plays a role in regulating insulin sensitivity and glucose metabolism, and deficiency is linked to an increased risk of metabolic syndrome and obesity. In urban areas where people spend a majority of their time indoors, vitamin D deficiency is more common, posing risks to metabolic health.

Sedentary Lifestyle Due to Urbanization

Urban environments often limit access to green spaces or opportunities for physical activity, contributing to sedentary lifestyles. Prolonged inactivity slows metabolic rate and contributes to weight gain and metabolic diseases. For example, studies show that physical inactivity leads to decreased insulin sensitivity and increased fat accumulation, both of which affect the body's ability to manage energy effectively.

Building Resilience to External Stressors

Environmental and lifestyle resilience refers to the body's ability to adapt to and counteract the effects of environmental stressors on metabolism. Building resilience involves making intentional choices that fortify the body's defenses against these stressors.

Strengthening the Immune System

A robust immune system can better manage and neutralize the effects of environmental toxins, pollutants, and pathogens. This can be achieved through a diet rich in antioxidants, vitamins, and minerals, which support immune cell function and reduce inflammation. Incorporating foods high in vitamin C , zinc, and antioxidants can strengthen the immune response and protect against oxidative stress induced by environmental factors.

Prioritizing a Balanced Diet

A balanced diet high in fiber, lean proteins, healthy fats, and complex carbohydrates provides essential nutrients that support metabolic health and resilience. Fiber-rich foods, for instance, support a healthy gut microbiome, which plays a role in metabolic regulation. Additionally, incorporating omega-3 fatty acids from sources like salmon, flaxseeds, and walnuts can help combat inflammation and improve insulin sensitivity.

Stress Management Techniques

Chronic stress elevates cortisol levels, which can negatively impact metabolism by promoting fat storage and increasing blood sugar levels. Stress-management techniques such as mindfulness meditation, deep breathing exercises, yoga, and spending time in nature can help lower cortisol levels, enhancing metabolic health and reducing the risk of insulin resistance and metabolic syndrome.

Quality Sleep for Optimal Recovery

Quality sleep is essential for metabolic resilience. Poor sleep disrupts circadian rhythms, increases hunger hormones, and impairs insulin sensitivity. Aim for 7-8 hours of uninterrupted sleep per night, and establish a consistent sleep routine to support your metabolism. Practices like limiting screen time before bed, creating a relaxing pre-sleep routine, and ensuring a dark, cool, and quiet sleep environment can enhance sleep quality and contribute to better metabolic health.

Increasing Physical Activity

Regular physical activity is one of the most effective ways to improve resilience to metabolic disruptions. Exercise enhances insulin sensitivity, reduces inflammation, and improves lipid metabolism, all of which are beneficial for maintaining metabolic health. Incorporating a mix of aerobic exercise, strength training, and flexibility exercises is ideal for building metabolic resilience. Exercise also promotes the production of endorphins, which help reduce stress and improve overall mood, indirectly supporting metabolic health.

Limiting Toxin Exposure

Minimizing exposure to environmental toxins can reduce their impact on metabolism. Practical steps include using natural or organic cleaning products, avoiding single-use plastics (which can leach chemicals like BPA), and choosing organic foods, when possible, to reduce pesticide exposure. These actions help limit the body's toxic burden, allowing the liver and kidneys to function optimally and maintain metabolic balance.

Practical Tips for a Healthier Lifestyle

Adopting a healthier lifestyle can strengthen metabolic health and improve resilience against environmental and lifestyle-related stressors. Here are some practical tips to help incorporate these habits effectively:

1. Eat a Diverse Diet

Consuming a variety of nutrient-dense foods supports metabolic health by providing a wide range of vitamins, minerals, and antioxidants. Aim to fill half your plate with colorful fruits and vegetables, include whole grains, and prioritize lean proteins. Limiting processed foods and sugars helps prevent metabolic disorders, while a balanced diet ensures sustained energy and stable blood sugar levels.

2. Stay Hydrated

Adequate hydration is essential for metabolic function, as water plays a key role in energy production, digestion, and the removal of toxins. Aim to drink at least eight glasses of water daily, or more if you are physically active or in a hot climate. Herbal teas and water-rich foods, such as cucumber, watermelon, and oranges, are also good sources of hydration.

3. Incorporate Regular Movement

Moving throughout the day prevents prolonged periods of inactivity that can lead to metabolic slowdown. Try to stand up, stretch, or take short walks every hour if you work a desk job. Consider taking the stairs instead of the elevator, walking to nearby destinations, or doing quick exercises like squats or jumping jacks to increase daily activity levels.

4. Practice Mindful Eating

Eating mindfully helps you become more attuned to hunger and fullness cues, preventing overeating and supporting a balanced metabolism. Focus on eating slowly, savoring each bite, and avoiding distractions, such as television or smartphones, during meals. This practice also enhances digestion and allows your body to process food more effectively.

5. Reduce Alcohol and Caffeine Intake

Excessive alcohol and caffeine consumption can disrupt sleep patterns, increase stress levels, and negatively affect metabolism. Limit alcohol to moderate levels and try to avoid caffeine in the afternoon to prevent sleep disturbances. If you rely on caffeine for energy, consider switching to lower-caffeine options like green tea or gradually reducing intake to support natural energy levels.

6. Engage in Stress-Relief Activities

Incorporate activities that relieve stress, such as journaling, gardening, or creative hobbies. Engaging in enjoyable activities fosters relaxation and enhances resilience to environmental stressors, benefiting both mental and metabolic health.

7. Optimize Your Environment for Wellness

Create a home environment that promotes relaxation and minimizes exposure to toxins. Use air purifiers to reduce indoor pollutants, choose non-toxic cleaning products, and reduce exposure to EMFs by keeping electronic devices out of the bedroom or placing them in airplane mode at night.

Conclusion

Environmental and lifestyle resilience is essential for maintaining metabolic health in today's world. By understanding the impact of environmental stressors on metabolism, building resilience, and implementing practical lifestyle changes, individuals can enhance their metabolic health and overall well-being. Simple, consistent efforts   like choosing nutrient-rich foods, managing stress, getting regular exercise, and minimizing toxin exposure build a strong foundation for lifelong metabolic resilience. Prioritizing these strategies can lead to sustained energy, improved mood, and greater health, empowering you to live your best life.

Chapter 10: Your Blueprint for Lasting Metabolic Health

Achieving lasting metabolic health is about more than just diet and exercise; it's a holistic approach that encompasses nutrition, physical activity, lifestyle choices, and mindset. This chapter provides a comprehensive guide to combining nutrition, exercise, and lifestyle practices to enhance metabolic function, helping you develop a personalized metabolic health plan for sustained energy and wellness. By creating a balanced approach, you'll set yourself up for long-term success and resilience against metabolic-related conditions.

Combining Nutrition, Exercise, and Lifestyle for Success

A successful approach to metabolic health integrates well-rounded nutrition, consistent exercise, and mindful lifestyle habits. Each of these components plays a crucial role in supporting the body's ability to efficiently process energy, manage weight, and sustain optimal function.

1. Nutrition as a Foundation for Metabolic Health

Proper nutrition is the cornerstone of metabolic health. It provides the body with essential nutrients, helps regulate blood sugar levels, and supports hormonal balance. Key strategies include:

- **Balanced Macronutrients:** Eating a diet that balances carbohydrates, proteins, and fats helps regulate blood sugar levels, control hunger, and improve insulin sensitivity. Complex carbohydrates, lean proteins, and healthy fats like those found in avocados, nuts, and olive oil are ideal for a balanced diet.

- **Fiber-Rich Foods:** High-fiber foods such as fruits, vegetables, legumes, and whole grains slow down digestion and stabilize blood sugar levels. Fiber also supports a healthy gut microbiome, which is essential for efficient metabolic function.

- **Anti-Inflammatory Foods:** Chronic inflammation can impair metabolism, so including anti-inflammatory foods, like berries, green leafy vegetables, turmeric, and fatty fish, can enhance metabolic health by reducing oxidative stress and inflammation.

- **Hydration:** Staying hydrated is critical, as water is essential for almost every metabolic function, including energy production and waste removal. Drinking adequate water supports cell function, improves digestion, and enhances physical and cognitive performance.

2. Exercise to Boost Metabolism

Physical activity is essential for improving metabolic health, as it increases calorie burn, supports cardiovascular function, and enhances insulin sensitivity. Different forms of exercise provide unique metabolic benefits:

- **Aerobic Exercise:** Activities such as walking, cycling, swimming, or jogging elevate heart rate and increase caloric burn, contributing to overall fat loss and improved cardiovascular health. Cardio exercises help maintain steady energy levels and boost endurance.

- **Strength Training:** Resistance training, including weight lifting and bodyweight exercises, builds muscle mass, which helps increase resting metabolic rate (RMR). A higher RMR means you burn more calories even at rest, making strength training a valuable tool for weight management.

- **High-Intensity Interval Training (HIIT):** HIIT involves short bursts of intense exercise followed by rest periods. It is highly effective for increasing metabolic rate, improving cardiovascular health, and enhancing fat oxidation. HIIT also improves insulin sensitivity and can be an efficient workout for those with limited time.

- **Flexibility and Mobility Exercises**: Practices like yoga and stretching improve muscle flexibility and joint mobility, reduce stress, and promote recovery. Yoga, in particular, combines physical activity with mindfulness, helping to reduce cortisol levels and support metabolic balance.

3. Lifestyle Factors and Mindfulness

Beyond diet and exercise, lifestyle factors such as stress management, sleep quality, and daily routines profoundly influence metabolic health. Incorporating healthy lifestyle habits can help sustain long-term metabolic balance:

- **Sleep Quality**: Sleep is when the body repairs and regenerates cells. Poor sleep disrupts hormones like cortisol, insulin, and ghrelin, which can lead to weight gain and insulin resistance. Prioritizing 7-8 hours of quality sleep each night is essential for hormonal balance and energy restoration.

- **Stress Management:** Chronic stress increases cortisol, which negatively affects metabolism by promoting fat storage and increasing blood sugar levels. Mindfulness practices like meditation, deep breathing, and journaling can lower cortisol and improve metabolic resilience.

- **Consistent Routine:** Establishing a consistent daily routine helps regulate the body's circadian rhythm, which supports metabolic health. Regular sleep patterns, meal times, and exercise routines align with your body's natural cycles, promoting stable energy levels and better digestion.

Developing a Personalized Metabolic Health Plan

Creating a personalized metabolic health plan involves assessing your individual needs, setting realistic goals, and making gradual, sustainable changes to your lifestyle. A customized plan empowers you to target specific areas of improvement, consider your preferences, and monitor progress for long-term success.

1.Setting Clear, Realistic Goals

Begin by defining clear goals. Are you focused on increasing energy, losing weight, reducing stress, or improving sleep? Setting specific, measurable, achievable, relevant, and time-bound (SMART) goals provides structure and motivation. For example, rather than aiming to "exercise more," set a goal to "do 30 minutes of strength training three times a week."

2. Assessing Current Habits and Identifying Areas for Improvement

Take stock of your current lifestyle. Evaluate your dietary habits, exercise routine, stress levels, and sleep quality. Identifying areas for improvement is key to creating an effective metabolic health plan. For example:

- **Nutrition Assessment:** Do you eat a balanced diet with whole foods, or do you rely heavily on processed foods? Consider introducing more whole foods, increasing your fiber intake, or balancing your macronutrients.

- **Exercise Patterns:** How active are you currently? If you're inactive, consider incorporating daily movement like short walks. For those already exercising, it may be beneficial to diversify activities or increase intensity.

- **Lifestyle Review:** How well do you manage stress? Are you getting sufficient sleep? Reflecting on these areas can help you make necessary adjustments.

3.Building a Flexible and Enjoyable Routine

A personalized plan should be flexible and enjoyable. Choose activities you enjoy, as this increases the likelihood of consistency. Flexibility also allows you to adapt to changes, such as a busy work schedule or travel, without feeling guilty or derailed. For instance:

- **Incorporate Enjoyable Foods:** Rather than restricting certain foods, focus on adding nutritious foods you enjoy. Find recipes that combine your favorite ingredients with healthy choices.

- **Explore Different Forms of Exercise**: If the gym isn't appealing, try dancing, hiking, or group sports. Choose activities that excite you and keep you motivated.

- **Mindful Adjustments:** Life can be unpredictable, so learning to make mindful adjustments is essential. If a workout or meal doesn't go as planned, practice self-compassion and resume your plan the next day.

4. Tracking Progress and Adjusting Goals as Needed

Regularly tracking your progress can help you stay motivated and identify any areas that need adjustment. Use a journal, app, or spreadsheet to log meals, exercise routines, sleep, and mood. Monitoring your energy levels, mood, and physical changes can also provide insight into how your plan affects your well-being. Adjust your goals if necessary, focusing on gradual improvements rather than immediate results.

Sustaining Energy and Wellness in Everyday Life

Long-term metabolic health is about integrating these changes into daily life in a way that is sustainable and enjoyable. Maintaining energy and wellness involves daily practices that support both mental and physical health, allowing you to build resilience and create a balanced lifestyle.

1. Prioritizing Consistency Over Perfection

Consistency is key for lasting metabolic health. Rather than aiming for perfection, focus on creating habits you can stick with over time. Daily choices, like opting for a salad over fast food or taking a walk during lunch breaks, add up over time and contribute to metabolic improvements. Even small, consistent efforts can lead to meaningful changes in metabolic health.

2. Creating a Balanced Mindset Toward Food and Exercise

Developing a positive relationship with food and exercise promotes mental well-being and prevents burnout. Avoid viewing food or exercise as punishment or reward, which can lead to unhealthy habits. Instead, see food as fuel and exercise as a way to enhance energy and support longevity. This balanced mindset fosters a healthy relationship with your body and motivates you to make choices that feel nurturing rather than restrictive.

3. Managing Stress in Everyday Situations

Stress management is a continuous process that can significantly impact metabolic health. Practice grounding techniques like deep breathing when stress arises, incorporate short breaks throughout the day, and allocate time for activities that bring joy. Even brief moments of mindfulness can help you stay grounded and support metabolic resilience.

4.Incorporating Movement Throughout the Day

While scheduled workouts are beneficial, incorporating movement throughout your day keeps energy levels steady and prevents metabolic stagnation. Simple changes, like using stairs instead of the elevator, standing up to stretch every hour, or taking short walks during breaks, can boost metabolism. Small actions add up and contribute to a more active lifestyle without needing a structured workout.

5.Optimizing Sleep Hygiene

Creating a sleep-friendly environment improves sleep quality, which is essential for metabolic function. Maintain a consistent sleep schedule, keep your bedroom dark and quiet, and limit screen exposure before bed. These practices help regulate the body's circadian rhythm, allowing for restorative sleep that supports metabolic processes and energy levels.

6.Celebrating   Progress   and   Practicing Self-Compassion

Lastly, acknowledge and celebrate the progress you make along your journey to lasting metabolic health. Practicing self-compassion can prevent feelings of frustration or guilt if you face setbacks. Remember that metabolic health is a lifelong commitment, and each day provides an opportunity to make choices that support your well-being. Embrace small wins, learn from challenges, and stay motivated by focusing on the positive impacts of your efforts.

Conclusion

Creating a blueprint for lasting metabolic health is about finding a balanced approach to nutrition, exercise, and lifestyle that works for you. By combining these elements into a personalized plan, you can improve metabolic function, sustain energy for daily vitality, and protect against metabolic-related conditions over time.

Notes.